Delicious Mediterranean Diet Cooking Plan

Stay Healthy and Fit with These New Recipes

Sofia Abagnale

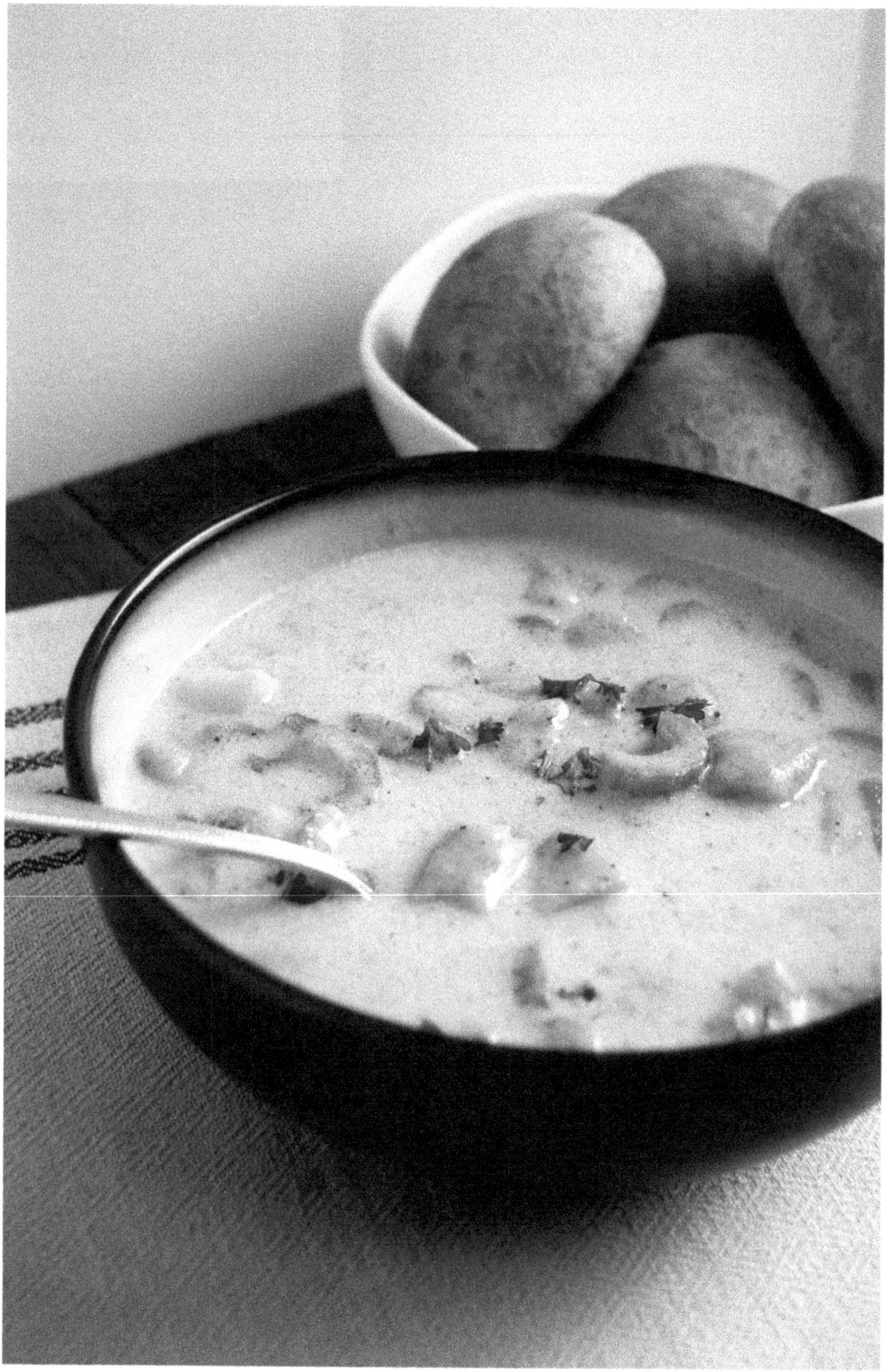

TABLE OF CONTENTS

Tortellini in brodo

Ingredients

- 50g of Parmesan cheese
- 150g of beef shank bones
- 75g of prosciutto di Parma
- olive oil
- 1 pinch of ground nutmeg
- 300g of free-range chicken thighs and drumsticks
- ½ of an onion
- 50g of mortadella di Bologna
- 1 stick of celery
- 1 carrot
- 200g tipo flour
- 300g of beef brisket
- 2 large free-range eggs
- 75g pf lean minced beef

Directions

1. Add carrots, chicken, unpeeled onion, celery, and a pinch of salt to a stockpot, cover with enough water.
2. Bring to boil, then cover, let simmer for 4 hours as you skim occasionally.

3. Blend the tipo flour with eggs in a food processor until soft but firm dough, wrap in Clingfilm, let rest for 30 minutes.

4. Heat a little olive oil, season the mince and fry until cooked through.

5. Drain any water, let cool.

6. Transfer to a blender with the prosciutto, mortadella, grated parmesan, and nutmeg. Blend until fine.

7. Divide the dough into 8 pieces. Use a pasta machine to roll out 1 piece into a long, flat, thin strip. Slice into 3cm squares.

8. Lightly dust a tray with flour.

9. Place a ¼ of a teaspoon of filling in the middle of a square of pasta.

10. Fold the pasta over into a triangle, and press to seal.

11. Repeat until you have used all the rolled-out dough.

12. Strain the stock and discard the meat and vegetables.

13. Taste and adjust the seasoning accordingly.

14. Bring to the boil, add tortellini and cook for about 3 minutes.

15. Serve and enjoy.

Summery pea soup with turmeric scallops

Ingredients

- ¼ teaspoon of ground turmeric
- 2 teaspoons of tamarind paste
- 1 bunch of spring onions
- 1 clove of garlic
- 175g of queen scallops
- 5cm piece of ginger
- ½ teaspoon of mustard seeds
- 1 fresh green Bird's-eye chili
- ½ a lime
- 1 teaspoon of cumin seeds
- 10 fresh curry leaves
- Groundnut oil
- 3 fresh curry leaves
- 800ml of organic vegetable
- 450g of fresh or frozen peas
- ½ teaspoon of jiggery

Directions

1. Toast the cumin seeds, add 2 tablespoons of oil with the spring onions, garlic, ginger, chili, and curry leaves.
2. Fry until sizzling, then pour in the stock and bring to the boil.
3. Add the peas, let simmer for 5 minutes.
4. Stir in the jiggery with the tamarind paste.
5. Season to taste.
6. Blender to purée until smooth. Set aside.
7. The heat 1 tablespoon of olive oil over a high heat.
8. Add the mustard seeds and stir continuously to form soup.
9. Mix in the turmeric with the curry leaves, scallops, fry briefly on each side, until beginning to brown.
10. Reheat the soup, taste, and adjust.
11. Serve and enjoy.

Ham ribollita

Ingredients

- 150g leftover ham
- 300g of cavolo Nero
- 1 onion
- 750ml of organic stock
- 2 cloves of garlic
- 1 x 400g tin of cannellini beans
- 2 sticks of celery
- 1 carrot
- Olive oil
- 2 teaspoons of fennel seeds
- 100g of spinach
- 1 x 400g tin of plum tomatoes

Directions

1. Heat a drizzle of olive oil over a medium heat.
2. Then, add celery, carrot, onion, garlic, and fennel seeds, and season.
3. Cook over low heat for 10 minutes covered, until golden brown, stirring regularly.
4. Mash most of the cannellini beans, add to the pan with the liquid from the tin, tomatoes, and the stock.

5. Let simmer for more 10 minutes.
6. Stir in chopped cavelo Nero, torn ham, and remaining beans, and spinach.
7. Simmer until the greens have cooked down.
8. Serve and enjoy.

Minestrone soup

Ingredients

- 2 x 400g tins of beans
- 100g of dried pasta
- 4 rashers of smoked streaky bacon
- Olive oil
- Parmesan cheese
- 1 clove of garlic
- 2 small onions
- Extra virgin olive oil
- 1 x 400g tin of quality plum tomatoes
- 2 fresh bay leaves
- 2 carrots
- 2 sticks of celery
- 2 large handfuls of seasonal greens
- 1 vegetable stock cube

Directions

1. Heat a large shallow casserole pan on a medium-high heat.
2. Sprinkle sliced bacon into the pan with 1 tablespoon of olive oil, stirring occasionally.

3. Add the chopped garlic, onion, and bay to the pan when the bacon turns golden.

4. Add chopped celery and carrots to the pan.

5. Remove and finely chop any tough stalks from your greens and add to the pan.

6. Let cook for 15 minutes, stirring regularly.

7. Pour in the tinned tomatoes with 1 tin's worth of water.

8. Add the beans together with the juice and a pinch of sea salt and black pepper.

9. Sprinkle greens into the pan, top with boiling water, then add the pasta.

10. Cover, let simmer for 15 minutes.

11. Taste, and adjust the seasoning accordingly.

12. Serve and enjoy with parmesan cheese.

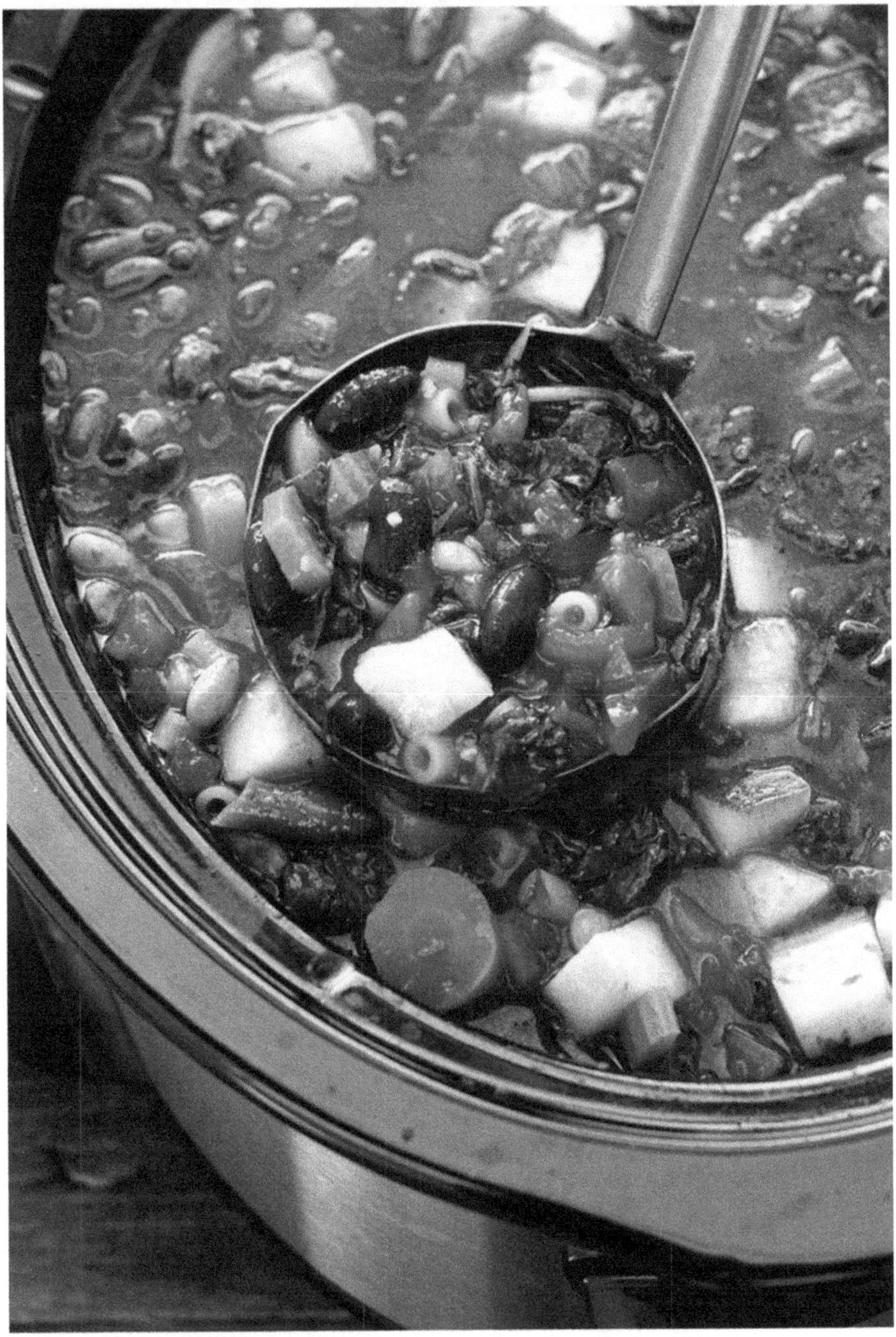

Spiced parsnips soup

Ingredients

- 800g of parsnips
- 4 sprigs of fresh coriander
- 1 onion
- 4 tablespoons of natural yoghurt
- 2 cloves of garlic
- 1.5 liters of organic vegetable stock
- 5cm piece of ginger
- Olive oil
- 4 uncooked poppadoms
- 1 teaspoon of cumin seeds
- Garam masala
- 200g of red split lentils

Directions

1. Start by preheating your oven ready to 350°F.
2. Place the parsnips and onions in a large pan over a medium heat with 1 tablespoon of olive oil.
3. Cook covered for 20 minutes, stirring occasionally.
4. Add the garlic together with the ginger, scatter over the cumin seeds, 1 teaspoon of garam masala and the lentils.
5. Cook for 5 more minutes.

6. Roughly snap in the uncooked poppadoms, stock, let simmer for 20 minutes.

7. Blanch reserved parsnips for 30 seconds in fast boiling water, drain and pat dry.

8. Season with sea salt.

9. Spread out in a single layer over a couple of oiled baking trays.

10. Let roast for 15 minutes.

11. Pick over the coriander leaves, sprinkle with a little garam masala, and top with the parsnip crisps.

12. Serve and enjoy.

Korean chicken hotpot

Ingredients

- 1 lime
- 150g of shiitake mushrooms
- 2 teaspoons of sesame oil
- 2 teaspoons of Korean chili paste
- 2 large carrots
- 250g of whole wheat noodles
- 1 bunch of spring onions
- 350g of firm silken tofu
- 2 teaspoons of sesame seeds
- 200g of kimchee
- 4 free-range chicken thighs
- 1 liter of organic chicken stock
- 1 teaspoon of low-salt soy sauce

Directions

1. Char the mushrooms in a casserole pan on a medium heat for 5 minutes, turning half way.
2. Remove the mushrooms to a plate, add the chicken and carrots to the pan.
3. Let cook for 10 minutes, stirring regularly.

4. Pour in the stock, bring to the boil, let simmer for 20 minutes.
5. Stir in the spring onions with mushrooms, tofu, soy sauce, and chili paste.
6. Let simmer again for 20 minutes.
7. Stir through the kimchee.
8. Cook the noodles according to the packet Directions, drain.
9. Toss with the sesame oil and seeds.
10. Taste the broth, and adjust the seasoning.
11. Serve and enjoy.

Playschool tomato soup

Ingredients

- 150g of pasta
- 2 x 400g tins of quality plum tomatoes
- 2 carrots
- 8 slices of sourdough
- 2 leeks
- 2 sticks of celery
- 2 onions
- Extra virgin olive oil
- 125g of mature Cheddar cheese
- 6 large ripe tomatoes
- 4 cloves of garlic
- Olive oil
- 1 organic chicken stock cube
- ½ a bunch of fresh basil

Directions

1. Preheat the oven to 375°F.
2. Toss all the vegetables and the tomatoes together in a deep roasting tray, season with season well with extra virgin olive oil.

3. Spread the vegetables into 1 layer, place in the oven for 40 minutes.
4. Bash pickled leaves to a paste, with a pinch of sea salt, until smooth.
5. Toss the basil stalks into the roasted vegetable, squeeze the garlic out of its skins into the tray, add tinned tomatoes and stock.
6. Bring to a boil over a medium heat.
7. Lower the heat, let simmer for about 15 minutes, or until thickened.
8. Remove the tray, pulse the soup until smooth.
9. Return the soup to the hob over a medium heat.
10. Then, season to taste and stir in the pasta.
11. Simmer for 5 minutes, or until the pasta is cooked.
12. Toast the bread, coarsely grate the cheese.
13. Place the hot soup into bowls, scatter over most of the cheese, stir through.
14. Top with a piece of toast, scatter over the remaining cheese, and finish with a drizzle of the basil oil.
15. Serve and enjoy.

Thai inspired vegetable broth

Ingredients

- 1 teaspoon of fish sauce
- 3 cloves of garlic
- 5cm piece of ginger
- 800ml of clear organic vegetable stock
- 1 small punned shiso cress
- 200g of mixed Asian greens
- 1 lime
- 2 spring onions
- 1 fresh red chili
- 1 teaspoon of soy sauce
- 5 sprigs of fresh Thai basil
- 1 stick of lemongrass
- 2-star anise

Directions

1. Bash the lemongrass on a chopping board with a rolling pin until it breaks open.
2. Add to a large saucepan together with the garlic, ginger, and star anise.
3. Pour in the vegetable stock in a pan over a high heat.

4. Bring let boil briefly, lower heat and gently simmer for 30 minutes.
5. Place in Asian veggies, let cook until they are wilted few minutes to cook time.
6. Serve the broth in deep bowls.
7. Seasoned with fish sauce and soy sauce, sprinkle with the herbs.
8. Serve and enjoy.

Hot and sour chicken broth

Ingredients

- 2 shallots
- 1 large handful of beansprouts
- Fish sauce
- 3 sticks of lemongrass
- 5cm of ginger
- 1.75 liters light organic chicken
- 2 cloves of garlic
- 3 limes
- 2 fresh red chilies
- ½ a bunch of fresh coriander
- Groundnut oil
- 1 bunch of spring onions
- 2 free-range chicken breasts

Directions

1. Gently sweat the shallots in a splash of oil until soft.
2. Place in the lemongrass together with the ginger, stock, most of the chili and garlic, and fry for 1 minute.
3. Add the chicken and simmer for 8 minutes, or until the chicken is cooked through.

4. Then, add a splash of fish sauce and squeeze in the lime juice.
5. Taste, and adjust seasoning with fish sauce, lime juice or chili.
6. Add the coriander, beansprouts, and spring onions.
7. Serve and enjoy.

Miso soup with tofu and cabbage

Ingredients

- ½ savoy cabbage
- 100g of silken tofu
- 750ml of organic chicken
- 1 carrot
- 3cm piece of ginger
- Low-salt soy sauce
- 2 cloves of garlic
- 2 tablespoons of miso paste
- 1 fresh red chili

Directions

1. Pour the stock into a pan, bring to a boil.
2. Add ginger, garlic, and chili to the stock, cover and simmer for 5 minutes.
3. Add carrots and cabbage to the pan, cover and simmer for 4 more minutes, or until the cabbage is wilted.
4. Then, stir in the miso paste and a good splash of soy sauce to taste.
5. Add the tofu and let it stand for a few minutes.
6. Serve and enjoy.

Asian inspired chicken rice balls and broth

Ingredients

- low-salt soy sauce
- 250g of mange tout
- 130g of brown rice
- 1 big bunch of coriander
- 6 spring onions
- 1 handful of beansprouts
- 4 skinless, boneless free-range chicken thighs
- 1 lime
- 2 packets of choi
- 1 stick of lemongrass
- 5cm piece of ginger
- 2 cloves of garlic
- 1 fresh red chili
- 4 kaffir lime leaves
- Sunflower oil
- 8 large raw king prawns
- 2½ tablespoons of miso paste

Directions

1. Start by cooking the rice according to the packet Directions.
2. Drain any excess water, let cool.
3. Place leaves in a food processor with the cooled rice except coriander leaves.
4. Add the onion, chicken, lemongrass, ginger, and garlic into the food processor with the kaffir lime leaves, blend until smooth.
5. Transfer the mixture onto a board.
6. Divide it into 16 pieces and roll each into a ball.
7. Place on a plate, chill, covered, until needed.
8. Place a large casserole pan over a medium-high heat.
9. Add a splash of sunflower oil. Fry the rice balls for 5 minutes, or until golden brown.
10. Add prawns to the pan, stir-fry for 1 minute.
11. Then, stir in the miso paste with boiling water, let simmer for 10 minutes.
12. Add Pak choi cut to 6 pieces with halved mange tout to the pan for the last 2 minutes.
13. Stir in the beansprouts for the last 30 seconds.
14. Season with a splash of soy sauce.
15. Serve and enjoy.

Watercress soup

Ingredients

- 400ml of organic stock
- 2 potatoes
- 3 bunches of watercress
- 2 onions
- Olive oil
- 2 cloves of garlic

Directions

1. In a large saucepan, heat bit of olive oil.
2. Sauté the potato with onion and garlic until the onions are translucent.
3. Add the stock and simmer until the potato is soft.
4. Add chopped watercress, let simmer for 4 minutes.
5. Liquidize the soup until smooth in a blender.
6. Serve and enjoy with a swirl of crème fraiche.

Simple noodle soup

Ingredients

- 300g of ready-prepared rice vermicelli
- 4 spring onions
- 1 splash of soy sauce
- 1 stick of lemongrass
- 2 cloves of garlic
- 225g of raw frozen prawns
- ½ a lime
- 2 fresh red chilies
- A few sprigs of fresh coriander
- 1 liter of organic chicken stock
- 1 bok choy

Directions

1. Bring the stock to boil in a large saucepan, lower heat, let simmer.
2. Add bok choy, prawns, spring onions, lemon grass, and garlic to the stock.
3. Cook for briefly, until the prawns have turned pink and the bok choy has wilted.
4. Divide the vermicelli between 4 bowls and ladle over the soup.

5. Then, scatter the chili with the coriander on top.

6. Season with soy and lime juice.

7. Serve and enjoy.

Fish soup

Ingredients

- 400g of prawns
- Olive oil
- 1 small bulb of fennel
- 1 leek
- Extra virgin olive oil
- 1 bunch of fresh thyme
- 3 sticks of celery
- 1 small glass of white wine
- 1 fresh red chili
- 4 cloves of garlic
- 4 tomatoes
- 440g of white fish

Directions

1. Begin by gently cooking over medium heat the fennel together with the leek, celery, most of the chili and the garlic in olive oil, until soft.
2. Add 1-liter water with the wine.
3. let boil, then reduce heat, simmer until vegetables are cooked.
4. Add the tomatoes together with the thyme and fish.

5. Once the fish turns opaque, add the prawns, let simmer for 2 minutes until prawns are cooked.
6. Season to taste.
7. Serve and enjoy with a drizzle of extra virgin olive oil and a scattering of fresh chili.

Parsnip, sage, and white bean soup

Ingredients

- 1 parsnip
- 1 onion
- 1 organic liter of chicken stock
- 2 large parsnips
- 2 sprigs of fresh sage
- Olive oil
- 1 x 420g tin of cannellini beans
- 1 sprig of fresh sage
- 1 fresh bay leaf

Directions

1. Heat 50ml of olive oil over a medium heat.
2. Cook the onion together with parsnips for 10 minutes, or until softened.
3. Add the bay leaf together with the beans, sage, and stock.
4. Season and let simmer for 15 minutes.
5. For the crispy parsnips, preheat the oven to 400°F.
6. Brush the parsnip slices and sage leaves with oil.
7. Then, bake for 10 minutes, or until crispy.

8. Remove and discard the bay leaf from the soup.

9. Beat with a stick blender until smooth.

10. Taste and adjust the seasoning accordingly.

11. Serve and enjoy with a drizzle of olive oil and the parsnip crisps on top.

Pumpkin and ginger soup

Ingredients

- 125ml of coconut milk
- 1kg of pumpkin
- 1-liter organic vegetable stock
- 2 shallots
- ½ tablespoon of chili powder
- 75g of ginger
- A few sprigs of fresh herbs
- Extra virgin olive oil
- 1 lime

Directions

1. Put the pumpkin together with the shallots, ginger, and bit of oil in a large saucepan, sauté until soft.
2. Add the stock with coconut milk and chili powder.
3. Season, bring to the boil, then let simmer for 40 minutes.
4. Transfer to a food processor and blend.
5. Serve and enjoy with the fresh herbs, lime juice and a splash of coconut milk.

Fresh tomato broth

Ingredients

- 1 x 2kg of whole free-range chicken
- 4 onions
- 20 large ripe mixed-color tomatoes
- 1 tablespoon of tomato purée
- 6 cloves of garlic
- 4 sticks of celery

Directions

1. Place the chicken together with the onions, garlic, celery, and tomatoes in a larger saucepan.
2. Then, add enough cold water to cover, bring to the boil over a high heat covered for 30 minutes.
3. Lower the heat when it begins to boil, let simmer over medium heat with the lid askew for 1 hour, or until the chicken is cooked through.
4. Only remove the chicken and put aside.
5. Sieve the soup and discard what is trapped.
6. Serve and enjoy with a drizzle of basil oil, herbs.

Super tasty miso broth

Ingredients

- 1 x 200g of skinless free-range chicken breast
- 1 handful of colorful curly kale
- 20g of dried porcini mushrooms
- 1 red onion
- 1 sheet of nori
- Groundnut oil
- Rice or white wine vinegar
- 150g of mixed exotic mushrooms
- 1 x 5cm piece of ginger
- 150g of mixed brown and wild rice
- 1 heaped teaspoon miso paste
- 800ml of chicken stock
- 6 radishes

Directions

1. Cook as per the package Directions. Drain.
2. Rehydrate the porcini in boiling water in a small bowl,
3. Place sliced onion, groundnut oil in a medium pan on a medium-high heat.
4. Cook briefly until dark golden, stirring occasionally.
5. Lower the heat to medium

6. Add the ginger with miso paste, porcini with soaking water, and stock.

7. Cover and simmer for 20 minutes.

8. Toss the radishes in a splash of vinegar with a small pinch of sea salt.

9. Stir through sliced chicken, torn kale, nori, broken mushroom.

10. Re-cover and cook for 4 minutes. Drain and divide the rice between bowls.

11. Season the broth according to your preference.

12. Serve and enjoy.

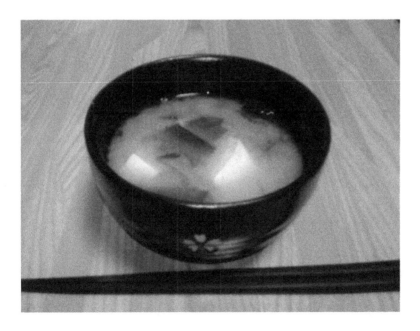

Roast carrot and fennel soup

Ingredients

- ½ teaspoon of dried yeast
- 1kg of carrots
- 250g of strong bread flour
- 1 onion
- 1 teaspoon of fennel seeds
- 1 teaspoon of sugar
- Olive oil
- 2 cloves of garlic
- 1.6 liters of organic vegetable stock
- 2 bulbs of fennel
- 100ml of single cream

Directions

1. Preheat your oven to 375°F.
2. Place carrots, onion, and fennel in a roasting dish, toss with 2 tablespoons of oil.
3. Roast for 20 minutes, add the unpeeled garlic cloves.
4. Stir vigorously and return to the oven for further 20 minutes, or until the vegetables are soft.
5. Discard garlic cloves.

6. Put the roasted vegetables in a large pan with the vegetable stock and bring to the boil.

7. Then, Simmer gently for 15 minutes, liquidize with a stick blender, until smooth.

8. Toast the fennel seeds in a dry frying pan briefly until fragrant.

9. Crush roughly, pour into a bowl with the flour and sea salt.

10. Dissolve the yeast and sugar in in hot water.

11. Add to the flour mixture with the olive oil and hot water and mix until dough foams, knead.

12. Divide the dough into 8 and roughly roll each one into a thin oval.

13. Stack them up, separating them with baking paper.

14. Heat a griddle pan until it's smoking hot, add the flatbreads.

15. Cook for briefly on each side, until charred and puffed up.

16. Serve and enjoy.

Chicken and vegetables soup

Ingredients

- 1 chicken carcass and bones
- 2 large onions
- 2 sticks of celery
- 1 leek
- Olive oil
- 2 sticks of celery
- 1 bunch of fresh flat-leaf parsley
- 5 black peppercorns
- 4 carrots
- 1 bunch of fresh flat-leaf parsley
- 2 courgette
- 200g of cooked chicken
- 100g of orzo
- 50g of frozen peas

Directions

1. Place in a large saucepan quartered onions, with chicken carcass, carrots, celery, peppercorns, and parsley.
2. Cover with cold water, season with a little sea salt.
3. Bring to the boil over a medium heat, skimming any froth off the surface.

4. Lower heat and simmer slowly for 3 hours when covered.

5. Strain the broth, let cool.

6. Add a splash of oil to a separate large saucepan and place over a medium heat.

7. Add onion, leek, celery, carrots, courgette, and parsley. Sauté for 5 minutes.

8. Stir in the orzo and stock, bring to a boil.

9. Lower the heat and simmer until the veggies are cooked.

10. Stir in the peas and chicken until heated through.

11. Season to taste.

12. Serve and enjoy.

Store cupboard lentil soup

Ingredients

- 1 organic vegetable stock cube
- 2 red onions
- ½ teaspoon dried thyme
- 200g of dried lentils
- Olive oil
- 2 carrots
- 1 x 410 g tin of cannellini beans
- 3 sticks celery
- ½ a dried chili
- 2 cloves garlic
- 6 rashers of smoked streaky bacon
- A few sprigs fresh flat-leaf parsley

Directions

1. Heat olive oil over a medium heat
2. Add the bacon and fry slowly until crispy, then crumble in the dried chili, dried thyme, carrot, celery, onion, and garlic.
3. Cook gently for about 15 minutes covered until all the vegetables are soft.
4. Add the lentils with a liter of water.

5. Bring to the boil and simmer until the lentils are soft.

6. Drain, then place in the cannellini beans.

7. Bring back to the boil and simmer for another 10 minutes.

8. Season with sea salt and black pepper.

9. Add into bowls and drizzle with extra virgin olive oil and the chopped parsley.

10. Serve and enjoy.

Ribollita

Ingredients

- 310g of cavelo Nero
- 1 bay leaf
- 2 large handfuls of good-quality stale bread
- 1 ripe tomato
- 1 pinch of dried red chili
- 1 small potato
- Extra virgin olive oil
- 1 x 400g tin of plum tomatoes
- 2 small red onions
- 2 carrots
- 3 cloves of garlic
- 3 sticks of celery
- Olive oil
- 1 pinch of ground fennel seeds

Directions

1. Place beans in a pan with bay leaf, tomatoes, and potatoes cook until the beans are tender. Drain and discard the bay leaf, tomato and potato. Reserve some bean water.
2. Heat a saucepan with a splash of olive oil.

3. Add the vegetables to the pan together with the ground fennel seeds and chili.

4. Sweat very slowly on a low heat with the lid just ajar for 20 minutes until soft.

5. Add the tomatoes and bring to a gentle simmer briefly.

6. Add the cooked and drained beans with a little of the reserved water, bring back to the boil.

7. Moisten and stir the bread.

8. Continue cooking for about 30 minutes.

9. Season with sea salt and black pepper.

10. Stir in extra virgin olive oil.

11. Serve and enjoy.

Corn chowder soup

Ingredients

- 1 medium potato, peeled and cut into little cubes
- 3 spring onions
- 1 medium onion
- Olive oil
- ½ teaspoon of dried thyme
- ¼ cup of fresh chives, chopped, or parsley
- 1 stalk celery
- 175g of frozen corn
- 1 tablespoon of plain flour
- 840ml of semi-skimmed milk

Directions

1. Heat the olive oil in a medium saucepan over a medium heat.
2. Add the celery, onion, and thyme.
3. Stir until vegetables start to brown.
4. Sprinkle the flour over the veggies and stir briefly.
5. Pour in the milk, then add the potato let boil, stirring the whole time so the soup, until the potatoes are tender in 10 minutes.

6. When the potatoes are tender, stir in the corn together with the spring onion and celery leaves.

7. Bring the soup back to the boil.

8. Serve and enjoy with crusty brown bread.

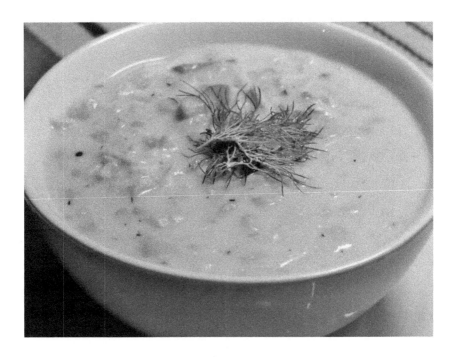

Roasted cauliflower and coconut soup

Ingredients

- 600g of cauliflower
- 1 x 400g tin of reduced-fat coconut milk
- 1 heaped teaspoon of ras el hanout
- 4 cloves of garlic
- 1 heaped teaspoon of ground cinnamon
- 3 tablespoons of chili oil
- Olive oil
- 1 handful of unsweetened coconut flakes
- 2 onions
- 600ml of vegetable stock

Directions

1. Preheat your oven to 350°F.
2. Place the onions, cauliflower in a roasting tray with the unpeeled garlic cloves and sprinkle with the cinnamon and ras el hanout.
3. Season, then drizzle with olive oil.
4. Toss, and place into the oven for 30 minutes, or until cooked through.

5. Scatter the coconut flakes on to a small tray, place briefly into the oven to toast.

6. When the vegetables are ready, remove the garlic cloves and scrape all the vegetables into a large saucepan.

7. Squeeze the garlic out of its skins and add to the mixture.

8. Pour in the coconut milk with stock, bring to the boil.

9. Lower the heat, let simmer for 5 minutes.

10. Blend the soup until creamy and smooth, adjust with water if too thick.

11. Taste and adjust the seasoning.

12. Serve and enjoy topped with the toasted coconut flakes and a drizzle of chili oil.

Chicken noodle soup

Ingredients

- 1 pinch of saffron
- Dry sherry
- Sweet ginger vinegar
- 200g of small carrots
- 100g of baby leeks
- 1 handful of fresh parsley stalks
- 300g of mixed fine pasta shapes
- 2 cloves of garlic
- 2-3 fresh bay leaves
- 200g of small onions
- 1 celery heart
- 5cm of piece of ginger
- 1 x 1.4kg of whole free-range chicken

Directions

1. Place celery, carrots, garlic, and onions into a very large saucepan with the chicken, bay leaves, and parsley stalks.
2. Season with sea salt and black pepper, then add enough water to cover the chicken.
3. Bring to the boil, lower the heat down, let simmer for 1 hour.

4. Empty the pan except for stock, then shred the chicken.
5. Bring the stock back to the boil and add a good splash of sherry with the saffron and a splash of ginger vinegar.
6. Add the pasta and continue to boil until the pasta is al dente.
7. Return the chicken and vegetables to the pan and simmer over low heat until warmed through.
8. Serve and enjoy.

Clear Asian noodle soup with prawns

Ingredients

- 1 carrot
- 100g of runner beans
- 2 large free-range eggs
- 250g of brown rice noodles
- 200g of cooked peeled king prawns
- 3cm piece of ginger
- 2 fresh hot Thai chilies
- 2 liters of organic chicken stock
- 2 tablespoons of sesame seeds
- 2 tablespoons of low-salt soy sauce
- 6 radishes
- 4 spring onions
- 2 cloves of garlic
- 2-star anise
- 6 cloves

Directions

1. Start by cooking the eggs in boiling water for 5 minutes.
2. Let cool under cold running water, peel and keep aside.

3. Cook the noodles according to the package Directions, drain, leave in a dish of cold water.

4. Add ginger and chili to a large pot together with the stock, unpeeled garlic cloves, soy sauce, star anise, and cloves.

5. Bring to a simmer, put off the heat, let infuse for 20 minutes.

6. Cook runner beans with carrot in a pan of boiling water for 2 minutes.

7. Drain, then plunge into cold water.

8. Strain the stock into a clean pot, return to a medium heat, then add sliced prawns.

9. Cook until just heated through.

10. Toast the onions and radishes with the sesame seeds in a dry frying pan.

11. Drain the rice noodles and divide between 4 bowls.

12. Sit the beans, carrot, and prawns on top.

13. Place over the broth and top with the radishes, spring onions, half an egg, and toasted sesame seeds.

14. Serve and enjoy.

Sweet potato, coconut, and cardamom soup

Ingredients

- 1 pinch of dried chili flakes
- 1 teaspoon of coriander seeds
- 3 green cardamom pods
- 2 jarred roasted peppers
- 800ml of organic vegetable
- 1 onion
- 100g of baby spinach
- 1 x 400ml tin of low-fat coconut milk
- 4cm piece of ginger
- 4 large poppadum
- 600g of sweet potato
- 2 cloves of garlic
- 3 tablespoons of groundnut oil
- 1 lemon

Directions

1. Crush the cardamom seeds in a mortar.

2. Heat groundnut oil over a low heat, then add the onion with a small pinch of sea salt let cook for 10 minutes in a large saucepan, stirring often.
3. Stir in the sweet potato together with the ginger, garlic, and crushed cardamom seeds.
4. Let cook for 2 minutes, then add the coconut milk.
5. Allow it to simmer for 2 minutes, stir in the stock.
6. Cover with a lid, and leave to simmer gently for 15 minutes.
7. Liquidize the soup in a blender until smooth.
8. Season with a pinch of salt and black pepper and a squeeze of lemon juice.
9. Heat groundnut oil in a frying pan, add crushed coriander seeds and chili flakes.
10. Let cook for 1 minute.
11. In a dry pan, toast the coconut flakes.
12. Add sliced peppers to the spices with the spinach.
13. Continue cooking until the spinach has wilted down.
14. Season and stir in the toasted coconut flakes.
15. Place the soup into bowls
16. Serve and enjoy topped with red pepper.

Beetroot and tomato borscht

Ingredients

- 2 celery stalks
- 1 clove of garlic
- 1.2 liters of organic beef stock
- 2 tablespoons of tomato purée
- A few sprigs of fresh dill
- 1 teaspoon of caster sugar
- 1 x 400g tin of plum tomatoes
- 2 large beetroot
- ½ of a small red cabbage
- 2 carrots
- 4 tablespoons of sour cream
- 1 red onion

Directions

1. Begin by pouring tomatoes into a large pan, stir in the onion with carrots, celery, garlic, beef stock, beetroot, tomato purée, and sugar.
2. Bring to the boil and simmer gently for 5 minutes.
3. Add the shredded cabbage, let simmer for another 30 minutes or so.
4. Blend the soup until smooth.

5. Serve and enjoy hot with swirls of the sour cream, then sprinkled with chopped dill.

Pistou soup

Ingredients

- 6 sprigs of fresh basil
- 60g of Parmesan cheese
- 1 onion
- 1 x 400g tin of borlotti beans
- 8 cloves of garlic
- 3 leeks
- 7 tablespoons of extra virgin olive oil
- 1 x 400g tin of cannellini beans
- 3 potatoes
- 3 carrots
- 1 stick of celery
- 3 courgettes
- 2 sprigs of fresh flat-leaf parsley
- 2 fresh bay leaves
- 250g of baby green beans
- 1 x 400g tin of chopped tomatoes
- 70g of small macaroni

Directions

1. Start by heating the olive oil over a medium heat.
2. Sauté the onion with garlic and leek for 5 minutes.

3. Add the potatoes, carrots, courgette, and celery, bay, green beans and chopped tomatoes.

4. Drain and add the beans.

5. Cover with water, then season, let simmer until the vegetables are tender.

6. Then, add the pasta and simmer until cooked. Regulate water as needed.

7. Place garlic, basil leaves, and sea salt in the mortar.

8. Pound until puréed, then finely grate in the Parmesan.

9. Muddle in the extra virgin olive oil to make a paste.

10. Serve and enjoy.

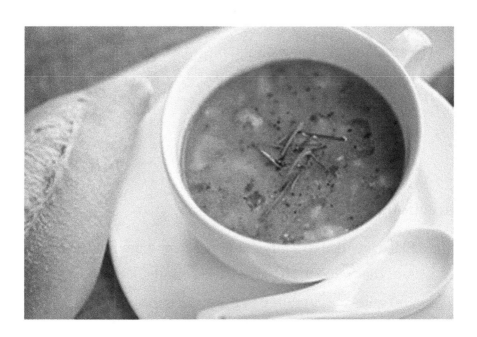

Celeriac and quince soup

Ingredients

- 2 banana shallots
- 1 teaspoon of ground cumin
- 2 cloves of garlic
- olive oil
- A few sprigs of fresh dill
- 1 organic chicken stock cube
- 1 teaspoon of sugar
- 1 quince
- 1 small handful of walnuts
- 1 tablespoon of crème fraiche
- 1 pinch of ground cinnamon
- 1 large celeriac

Directions

1. Place olive oil to a large pan, put over a medium-low heat.
2. Add the celeriac, shallots, garlic, cumin, cinnamon, sugar, and quince, crumbling in the stock cube.
3. Let cook gently for 25 minutes, stirring occasionally.
4. Add in enough boiling water to cover the vegetables once all vegetables have softened.

5. Uncover and let simmer for 25 minutes, or until the vegetables are cooked through.

6. Blend to your preferred consistency.

7. Roughly chop the walnuts and toast in a little butter.

8. Then, top the soup with a swirl of crème fraiche, a little picked dill and a handful of chopped toasted walnuts.

9. Serve and enjoy.

Red lentil, sweet potato, and coconut soup

Ingredients

- ½ a bunch of fresh coriander
- 1 liter of organic vegetable stock
- 750g of sweet potatoes
- 1 x 400g tin of light coconut milk
- 2 red onions
- 125g of red lentils
- ½ tablespoon of cumin seeds
- 1 teaspoon of ground coriander
- Olive oil
- 1 lemon
- 4 cloves of garlic
- 1 fresh red chili

Directions

1. Preheat the oven to 350°F.
2. Place sweet potatoes with onion wedges in a roasting tray in an even manner.
3. Sprinkle over the cumin seeds with ground coriander and a pinch of sea salt and black pepper.

4. Then, drizzle with oil, toss to coat.
5. Place in the oven for 45 minutes, or until golden.
6. Place a large saucepan over a medium-low heat and pour in a lug of oil.
7. Sauté the garlic together with the chili and coriander stalks briefly, until lightly golden.
8. Add the red lentils to the pan.
9. Stir to coat, then pour in the hot stock with coconut milk.
10. Raise the heat, let boil, then simmer.
11. Cook the lentils for 20 minutes.
12. Remove from the oven when veggies are ready, spoon into the pan.
13. Add most of the coriander leaves, then blend the soup until creamy with some little texture.
14. Taste and adjust the seasoning with lemon juice.
15. Serve and enjoy with coriander leaves.

Spiced parsnip and lentil soup with chili oil

Ingredients

- 3 tablespoons of groundnut oil
- 1 small smoked ham hock
- A few sprigs of fresh mint
- 1 onion
- 1 garlic clove
- Fat-free Greek yoghurt
- 3cm piece of ginger
- 400g of parsnips
- Olive oil
- 250g of red lentils
- 2 red chilies
- 2 tablespoons of Rogan paste
- 1.6 liters of organic vegetable stock

Directions

1. Soak the ham hock in cold water overnight.
2. Drain and place it in a saucepan.
3. Cover with cold water, bring it to the boil.
4. Lower the heat, let simmer for 2 hours.

5. Drain again, and set aside.

6. Place the groundnut oil in a pan over a very low heat.

7. Add sliced garlic and chilies to the pan, warm for 5 minutes.

8. Heat olive oil in a large pan, then add the onion.

9. let cook gently for 5 minutes, stirring frequently.

10. Add the parsnips together with the rogan paste and ginger, let cook for 5 minutes.

11. Add the lentils, stock, and the ham hock, bring to the boil.

12. Simmer for about 30 minutes, until the lentils soften.

13. Remove and discard the ham bone and liquidize the soup until smooth.

14. Return any lean ham to the saucepan and reheat.

15. Shred the mint leaves and serve scattered on top of the soup with a dollop of yoghurt.

16. Serve and enjoy.

Caldo Verde

Ingredients

- Paprika
- 1 large onion
- Extra virgin olive oil
- 2 cloves of garlic
- 300g of kale
- 150g of chorizo
- 700g of potatoes

Directions

1. Start by heating 4 tablespoons of oil in over medium heat.
2. Fry the onion with garlic for 5 minutes, or till soft.
3. Stir in the potatoes, then season with sea salt, let cook for 5 minutes.
4. Add water, then simmer for 20 minutes.
5. Then, mash the potatoes into the liquid to produce a smooth purée.
6. Add the kale, let simmer for 5 minutes.
7. Heat 1 tablespoon of oil in a frying pan over medium heat.
8. Fry the chorizo slices, sprinkling with paprika in the pan for 4 minutes.

9. Add the chorizo to the soup.
10. Place the soup into bowls and season with freshly ground black pepper.
11. Serve and enjoy with slices of corn bread.

Baked potato soup

Ingredients

- Sour cream
- 3 large baking potatoes
- 1 Parmesan rind
- 40g of butter
- 1.5 liters of organic chicken
- 1 small bunch of fresh chives
- 1 onion

Directions

1. Preheat the oven to 360°F.
2. Prick cleaned potatoes with a fork and wrap in foil.
3. Place on a rack in the middle of the oven, let cook for about 1 hour 15 minutes.
4. Remove, when cool enough, cut into quarters. Let cool completely.
5. Melt butter over a medium-low heat, add and cook diced onion for 10 minutes.
6. Add the potato with Parmesan rind to the pan.
7. Season, and cook for 5 minutes.
8. Add the stock, bring to the boil.
9. Lower the heat, let simmer for 30 minutes.

10. Remove, purée the soup until smooth without the rind.

11. Return to the pan.

12. Taste, and adjust the seasoning.

13. Serve and enjoy with a dollop of sour cream, snipped chives and a pinch of black pepper.

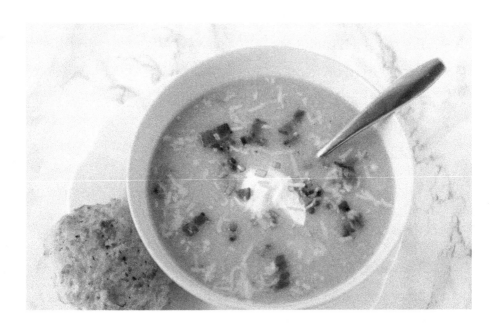

Caprese soup

Ingredients

- 1½ tablespoons red wine vinegar
- 50g of basil leaves
- 1 bulb of garlic
- 4 slices of sourdough bread
- 1kg of mixed tomatoes
- Extra virgin olive oil
- 2 x 125g of balls of buffalo mozzarella
- 4 sun-dried tomatoes in oil
- 1 tablespoon of soft brown sugar

Directions

1. Preheat the oven ready to 400°F.
2. Place cut garlic in a large roasting tray with the tomatoes.
3. Drizzle with 1 tablespoon of olive oil.
4. Let roast in the oven for 25 minutes, or until the tomatoes have burst.
5. Let cool totally.
6. Squeeze and roasted garlic into a blender with the roasted tomatoes, sugar, basil, sun-dried tomatoes, vinegar, and 3 tablespoons of oil.
7. Blend until smooth, then transfer to a jug.

8. Heat a griddle pan and chargrill the sourdough on both sides.

9. Serve and enjoy with half a torn mozzarella ball in the center topping with basil leaves and cracked black pepper.

Goulash soup

Ingredients

- 1 tablespoon of tomato purée
- 250g of onions
- 2 cloves of garlic
- ½ tablespoon of caraway seeds
- 200g of potatoes
- 1 green pepper
- 2 tomatoes
- Sour cream
- A few sprigs of fresh marjoram
- Extra virgin olive oil
- 500g of beef shin
- Red wine vinegar
- 1 tablespoon paprika
- 1½ liters of organic beef stock

Directions

1. Place a splash of extra olive oil in a large pan.
2. Sauté the onions with garlic and pepper until softened.
3. Add the beef and continue to cook until the meat is browned and the vegetables are cooked.
4. Then, stir in the paprika, let cook for 2 minutes.

5. Add the beef stock.

6. Bring to the boil until reduced by half.

7. Add the marjoram together with the tomatoes, the tomato purée, caraway seeds, a splash of vinegar, season well.

8. Add enough stock to cover, let simmer until the meat and vegetables are tender, in 2 hours.

9. Add diced potatoes, with the remaining stock.

10. Let simmer until the potatoes are cooked.

11. Serve and enjoy with a dollop of sour cream.

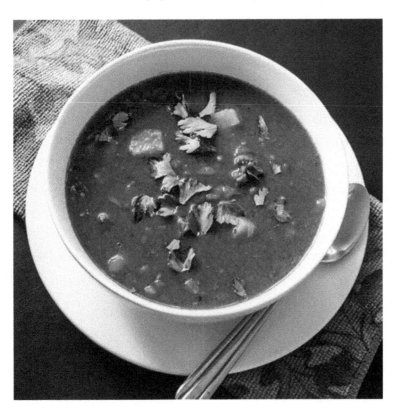

Costa Rican black bean soup

Ingredients

- 4 large free-range eggs
- 3 red onions
- 1 tablespoon of red wine vinegar
- ½ a bunch of fresh thyme
- 2 cloves of garlic
- 2 sticks of celery
- Extra virgin olive oil
- 2 x 400g tins of black beans
- 2 fresh bay leaves
- 1 green pepper
- 4 corn of tortillas
- 1 red pepper
- 2 fresh red chilies
- ½ a bunch of fresh coriander
- Olive oil

Directions

1. Drizzle olive oil in a large saucepan over a medium-low heat.
2. Add 2/3 of chopped onion, garlic, celery, coriander stalks, and peppers and thyme leaves to the pan.

3. Add ½ of chili, gently sauté the veggies for 15 minutes.
4. Place black beans with their liquid, bay leaves, and boiling water.
5. Raise the heat and bring to the boil.
6. Season well.
7. Lower the heat, let simmer, for 30 minutes covered, or until creamy.
8. Then, crack the eggs directly into the soup over reduced the heat.
9. Leave the eggs to poach in the soup for 5 minutes.
10. Add chopped coriander with remaining chopped onion, red wine vinegar, and a few tablespoons of extra virgin olive oil. Mix well.
11. Serve and enjoy with black bean soup.

Mulligatawny soup

Ingredients

- 1 x 400g tin of chopped tomatoes
- 1 large onion
- 2 cloves of garlic
- 500g leftover of free-range turkey
- 750ml of hot organic chicken
- 1 carrot
- 300g of butternut squash
- 300g of basmati rice
- 1 thumb-sized piece of ginger
- 1 tablespoon of tomato purée
- 1 tablespoon of olive oil
- a few sprigs of fresh coriander
- 1 dried red chili
- 1 tablespoon of curry paste

Directions

1. Firstly, heat olive oil in a large saucepan over a medium heat.
2. Add the onion together with the garlic, carrot, ginger, and dried chili.

3. Cover, and cook, stirring occasionally, until all the vegetables are soft and lightly golden.

4. Then, add the butternut squash with tomato purée and curry paste, shred in the turkey, and stir to coat.

5. Add the chopped tomatoes.

6. Season with sea salt and black pepper.

7. Pour in the hot stock and bring to the boil.

8. Lower heat and let simmer for 15 minutes.

9. Add the basmati rice and simmer for a further 10 minutes.

10. Serve and enjoy garnished with coriander leaves.

Turkey and coconut milk soup

Ingredients

- 100g of oyster mushrooms
- 3 Thai shallots
- 200g of cooked, skinless turkey
- 2 bird's-eye chilies
- 1 thumb-sized piece of galangal or ginger
- 3 kaffir lime leaves
- 2 tablespoons of fish sauce
- 3 coriander roots
- A few sprigs of fresh coriander
- 2 lemongrass stalks
- 500 ml organic turkey
- 1 x 400ml tin of light coconut milk
- 1 teaspoon of palm
- 1/2 lime

Directions

1. Add the stock with the coconut milk to a large saucepan.
2. Bring to the boil, then turn down the heat.
3. Add the sugar together with the chilies, lime leaves, lemongrass, shallots, galangal or ginger, and coriander roots.

4. Season and simmer gently for 5 minutes.
5. Add torn mushroom and shredded turkey to the pan.
6. Lower the heat to low.
7. Simmer for 3 minutes, and add the fish sauce and lime juice.
8. Serve and enjoy hot with some coriander leaves.

Roasted carrot and fennel soup

Ingredients

- ½ teaspoon of dried yeast
- 1 teaspoon of sugar
- 1 teaspoon of fennel seeds
- 1kg of carrots
- 100ml of single cream
- 250g of strong bread flour
- 1 onion
- 2 bulbs of fennel
- Olive oil
- 2 cloves of garlic
- 1.6 liters of organic vegetable stock

Directions

1. Preheat the oven to 375°F.
2. Place sliced carrots, onion, and fennel in a roasting dish, and toss bit of oil.
3. Let roast for 20 minutes, add the unpeeled garlic cloves.
4. Stir, return to the oven for 20 more minutes, or until the vegetables are browned.
5. Remove, discard the papery skins from the garlic cloves.

6. Put the roasted veggies in a large pan with the vegetable stock, bring to the boil.
7. Then, simmer for 15 minutes, then liquidize with a stick blender, until completely smooth.
8. Toast the fennel seeds in a dry frying pan for 30 seconds.
9. Crush roughly with mortar, then pour into a bowl with the flour and sea salt.
10. Dissolve the yeast and sugar in hot water.
11. Add to the flour mixture with the oil and hot water, mix until dough foams. Knead for 5 minutes.
12. Place the dough into an oiled bowl, cover with oiled Clingfilm and set aside to rise.
13. Divide the dough into 8, roll each one into a thin oval.
14. Stack up, separating them with baking paper.
15. Heat a griddle pan until very hot.
16. Add the flatbreads let cook briefly on each side, until charred.
17. Serve and enjoy with a swirl of cream, a scattering of herby fennel tops.

Steaming ramen

Ingredients

- 8 chicken wings
- 1 handful of pork bones
- 200ml of low-salt soy sauce
- 2 sheets of wakame seaweed
- 750g of pork belly
- 2 thumb-sized pieces of ginger
- Sesame oil
- 1 thumb-sized piece of ginger
- 1 splash of mirin
- 1 heaped tablespoon of miso paste
- 400g of baby spinach
- 500g of dried soba
- 8 tablespoons of kimchee
- 8 small handfuls of beansprouts
- 4-star anise
- 8 spring onions
- 7 garlic
- 2 fresh red chilies
- Chili oil
- 4 large free-range eggs

Directions

1. Boil the eggs for 5 minutes.
2. Pour the soy sauce, mirin, and star anise, with water into a small pan.
3. Boil ginger and garlic, remove from the heat, then, pour the mixture into a sandwich bag with the eggs.
4. Place in refrigerator for 6 hours, then drain.
5. Preheat the oven to 400°F.
6. Place chicken wings together with the pork bones into a large casserole pan.
7. Bash, add the unpeeled ginger and garlic.
8. Toss with a good drizzle of sesame oil.
9. Place the pork skin on a baking tray, bake for around 40 minutes.
10. Cover pork belly and miso with water, bring to the boil.
11. Simmer over low heat for 3 hours, or until the pork belly is tender, skimming occasionally.
12. Lift the pork belly onto a tray and put aside.
13. Sieve the broth and pour back into the pan. Return to the heat and reduce the liquid down.
14. Place a large colander over the pan and steam the spinach until wilted.
15. In another separate pan, cook the noodles according to packet Directions, drain.
16. Divide between 8 large warm bowls with the beansprouts and spinach.

17. Taste the broth and adjust the seasoning.

18. Tear over the seaweed and divide up the kimchee.

19. Serve and enjoy drizzle with chili oil.

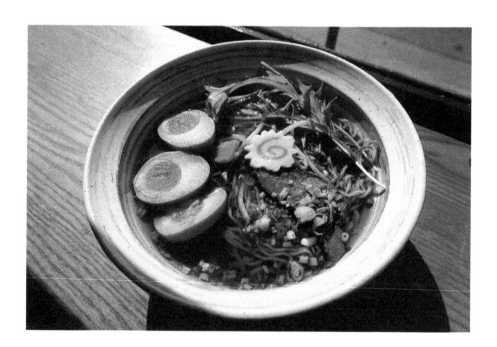

Apple and celeriac soup

Ingredients

- 200ml of crème fraiche
- 4 tablespoon of olive oil
- 2 onions
- 2 liters of vegetable stock
- A few sage leaves
- 1 celery stalk
- Toasted hazelnuts
- 1 celeriac
- 4 apples
- A few sprigs of thyme

Directions

1. Heat half of the olive oil in a large pan.
2. Add sliced onions, celery, let cook over a medium heat for 10 minutes until soft.
3. Add Chopped celeriac, apples, and thyme leaves to the pan, let cook for 2 to 3 minutes.
4. Add the stock and season.
5. Let simmer over a low heat for 30 minutes.
6. Remove, and blend until smooth.
7. Then, stir in half the crème fraiche.

8. Heat the remaining olive oil in a pan, fry the sage leaves until crispy.

9. Spoon the soup into bowls and top with the remaining crème fraiche.

10. Serve and enjoy with a drizzle of extra virgin olive oil, sprinkled with the crispy sage leaves and hazelnuts

Roasted tomatoes and bread soup

Ingredients

- 2kg of ripe tomatoes
- ½ a bulb of garlic
- 2 red onions
- 1 pinch of dried oregano
- Olive oil
- 1 liter of organic vegetable stock
- A few sprigs of fresh basil
- 1 x 280g of ciabatta loaf
- Red wine vinegar
- Extra virgin olive oil

Directions

1. Preheat the oven to 400°F.
2. Place cut tomatoes on a large roasting tray.
3. Scatter garlic bulbs and wedges of onions into the tray.
4. Sprinkle with oregano.
5. Season with sea salt and black pepper.
6. Drizzle with oil, then let roast for 1 hour, or until the tomatoes sticky.

7. Pour in the stock, roughly chop and add the basil stalks with most of the leaves.

8. Tear 1 half of ciabatta loaf into the soup.

9. Bring to the boil, simmer for 10 minutes.

10. Heat a griddle pan to high.

11. Slice the remaining ciabatta and griddle until lightly charred on both sides.

12. Add 1 splash of red wine vinegar to the soup.

13. Blend until fairly smooth.

14. Ladle into bowls, drizzle with extra virgin olive oil and scatter with the

15. remaining basil leaves.

16. Serve and enjoy with griddled ciabatta on the side.

Garden glut soup

Ingredients

- 1 organic vegetable stock cube
- 1 medium onion
- 100g of podded fresh peas
- A2 sticks of celery
- a few sprigs of fresh mint
- 1 medium leek
- 200g of baby spinach
- 2 cloves of garlic
- Olive oil
- 3 medium potatoes

Directions

1. Combine chopped onion, celery, garlic, and leek in a small bowel.
2. Place a large pot on a medium heat with 2 tablespoons of olive oil.
3. When hot, add vegetables the in the small bowl, lower the heat and cook with the lid askew for 10 to 15 minutes, stirring occasionally.
4. Place chopped potatoes, courgette in a bowl.
5. Fill and boil the kettle.

6. Add the potatoes, courgettes, once the vegetables are cooked, with a tiny pinch of sea salt and black pepper.
7. Crumble the stock cube into a measuring jug.
8. Top up the boiling water and stir until dissolved.
9. Pour the hot stock into the pot.
10. Raise the heat to high and bring to the boil.
11. Cook over low heat for 15 to 20 minutes or until the potato is cooked through.
12. Add the peas with spinach and cook for 4 more minutes.
13. Remove the pot to a heatproof surface, let rest.
14. Blend until smooth.
15. Ladle the soup into bowls and sprinkle over the mint.
16. Serve and enjoy.

Asian noodles broth with fish

Ingredients

- 2 fresh red chilies
- 250g of fresh egg noodles
- 2 limes, juice
- Sea salt
- Low-salt soy sauce
- 220g can of water shell nuts
- Freshly ground black pepper
- Sesame oil
- Vegetable oil
- 2 cloves garlic
- 1 small bunch fresh coriander
- 1 thumb-sized piece of fresh ginger
- 100g of mange tout
- 1 liter of organic fish
- 500g of sole fillets

Directions

1. Bring a pan of salted water to the boil.
2. Place in and cook the noodles as instructed on the pack.
3. Drain the noodles in a colander, toss in a little sesame oil.
4. Divide the noodles between four serving bowls.

5. Heat a large frying pan over a medium heat.

6. Add a splash of vegetable oil.

7. Stir-fry the garlic together with the ginger, mange tout, water shell nuts, and half the chilies for 2 minutes.

8. Add the hot stock and bring to the boil.

9. Place in the sole pieces, cook for a minute.

10. Season generously with soy sauce and black pepper.

11. Serve and enjoy.

Brown Windsor soup with pearl barley

Ingredients

- 1 tablespoon of plain flour
- 1 large knob of unsalted butter
- Olive oil
- 2 liters of organic beef stock
- 1 fresh bay leaf
- 500g of diced stewing steak
- 1 tablespoon of Marmite
- 2 carrots
- 150g of pearl barley
- 1 splash of Worcestershire sauce
- 1 sprig of fresh rosemary
- 1 red onion
- 3 sticks of celery

Directions

1. Melt the butter in a large pan over a medium heat.
2. Add a splash of olive oil with the steak, and lightly brown the meat.
3. Stir in the Marmite with the Worcestershire sauce.

4. Raise the heat to high and keep stirring until all the liquid has evaporated.

5. Add carrots together with the onions, bay leaf, rosemary sprig, and celery, cook over a low heat covered until soft.

6. Stir in the flour, pour in the stock.

7. Season well with sea salt and black pepper.

8. Bring to the boil, lower the heat to let simmer.

9. Add the pearl barley, let cook gently for 1 hour.

10. Remove, then discard the rosemary sprig with bay leaf.

11. Whisk the soup to thicken.

12. Serve and enjoy with hunks of soda bread.

Chicken garden soup

Ingredients

- A few sprigs of fresh flat-leaf parsley
- 2 onions
- 200g of baby spinach
- 6 carrots
- 2 handfuls of seasonal greens
- 6 sticks of celery
- 1 lemon
- 1 large knob of unsalted butter
- 2 fresh bay leaves
- 4 shallots
- 4 whole peppercorns
- 2 cloves of garlic
- 1 free-range of roast chicken carcass
- Olive oil

Directions

1. Put chopped onions, carrots, celery, bay leaves, peppercorns, chicken carcass, and a pinch of salt in a bowl.
2. Fill the pan with cold water, then place on a high heat and bring to the boil.

3. Lower the heat, let a simmer and cook for 1 hour, skimming off any scum.

4. About 20 minutes before the stock is ready, crack on with the base of the soup.

5. Place the butter with 1 tablespoon of oil in a separate large pan on a low heat.

6. Add the garlic together with the shallots and parsley stalks, let cook for 10 minutes.

7. Add the carrots with celery, cook for a further 5 minutes.

8. When the stock is ready, remove the chicken carcass with any remaining pieces of meat and leave to one side. Throw the carcass.

9. Strain the stock through a sieve into the veggie pan.

10. Bring to the boil, then reduce heat, simmer for 20 minutes.

11. Add the seasonal greens, cook for 10 minutes.

12. Add the spinach in the last minute.

13. Divide between bowls and top with any leftover shredded chicken.

14. Serve and enjoy sprinkled with parsley leaves and black pepper.

Chunky squash and chickpea soup

Ingredients

- 1 dried red chili
- Sea salt
- A few sprigs of fresh mint
- Olive oil
- 2 sticks celery
- 1 tablespoon of cumin seeds
- Harissa paste
- 2 lemons, zest
- 3 cloves garlic
- A few sprigs of fresh flat-leaf parsley
- 1 butternut squash
- 2 small red onions
- Extra virgin olive oil
- 1.5 liters of organic chicken
- 2 x 400g of tinned chickpeas
- 50g of almond flakes
- ½ tablespoon of fennel seeds
- ½ tablespoon of sesame seeds
- ½ tablespoon of poppy seeds
- Freshly ground black pepper

Directions

1. Begin by preheating your oven ready to 400°F.
2. Place the squash together with the cumin, and crumbled chili on to a baking tray.
3. Drizzle with olive oil, mix together and place in the preheated oven.
4. Roast for 45 minutes until the squash is cooked through.
5. Heat a large saucepan once the squash is roasted, pour in a splash of oil.
6. Add the celery together with the garlic, parsley stalks, and 2/3 of the onion, cook gently until softened, covered.
7. Place in the roasted squash and let it sweat for a few minutes
8. Pour in the stock. Bring to the boil.
9. Let simmer for 15 minutes over low heat.
10. Add the chickpeas and simmer for 15 minutes more.
11. Toast the reserved squash seeds with the almond flakes, fennel, sesame, and poppy seeds in a little olive oil until all colored.
12. Season, then blend briefly to thickens.
13. Mix lemon zest together with the chopped parsley leaves, and mint leaves.
14. Chop the remaining onion until it's really fine, add to zesty mixture, mix.
15. Spoon half a teaspoon of harissa paste into each bowl.

16. Divide the zesty herb mixture between the bowls and ladle over the soup.

17. Stir each bowl with a spoon

18. Serve and enjoy with the toasted seeds and almonds

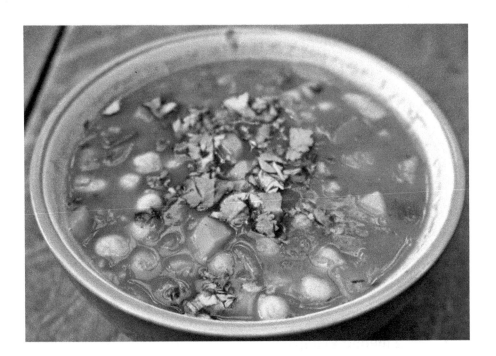

Summertime pasta salad with tomatoes, corn, and jalapeno pesto

Ingredients

- ½ teaspoon of salt
- ½ cup of olive oil
- 1 can of black beans
- 1-pint of cherry tomatoes
- 1 ear of fresh corn, shucked
- Freshly ground black pepper
- ½ pound of whole grain bow-tie pasta
- ¾ cup crumbled feta
- 1 cup of fresh parsley
- 1 cup of cilantro
- ½ cup of pepitas
- 2 medium jalapeños
- 1 medium lemon, juiced
- 1 medium garlic clove

Directions

1. Bring a large pot of salted water to boil.
2. Cook the pasta according to package directions.
3. Drain, reserve some cooking water.
4. Toast the pepitas in a small skillet over medium heat, stirring frequently, until lightly golden on the edges.
5. Combine the herbs, jalapeño, lemon, garlic, and salt in a food processor.
6. Pour in the pepitas.
7. Pulse while drizzling in the olive oil until the mixture is well blended.
8. Pour enough pesto into the pasta to lightly coat it once tossed.
9. Add a small splash of pasta cooking water and toss well.
10. Transfer the pasta to a large serving bowl.
11. Add the drained black beans, sliced cherry tomatoes, fresh corn and feta.
12. Serve and enjoy.

Tropical mango spring rolls with avocado cilantro dipping sauce

Ingredients

- ½ cup of lightly packed fresh cilantro
- 2 ripe mangos
- ⅓ cup of water
- ½ teaspoon of salt
- 1 large red bell pepper
- 2 jalapeños
- 4 green onions
- 7 round of rice papers
- 3 cups of arugula
- 2 ripe avocados, diced
- ⅓ cup of lime juice

Directions

1. Fill a shallow pan with warm water. Fold a lint-free tea towel in half and place it next to the dish.
2. Place one rice paper in the water and let it rest for 20 seconds. Carefully lay it flat on the towel.
3. Cover the lower third of the paper with chopped arugula.
4. Top with 4 slices of mango down the length of the greens.

5. Then, followed by several slices of bell pepper and jalapeño, sprinkle of green onions.

6. Fold over one long side to enclose the filling, then fold over the short sides, roll it up. Repeat with remaining ingredients.

7. Combine the avocado, lime juice, water, cilantro, and salt in a small food processor.

8. Purée until smooth and transfer to a small serving bowl.

9. Serve and enjoy.

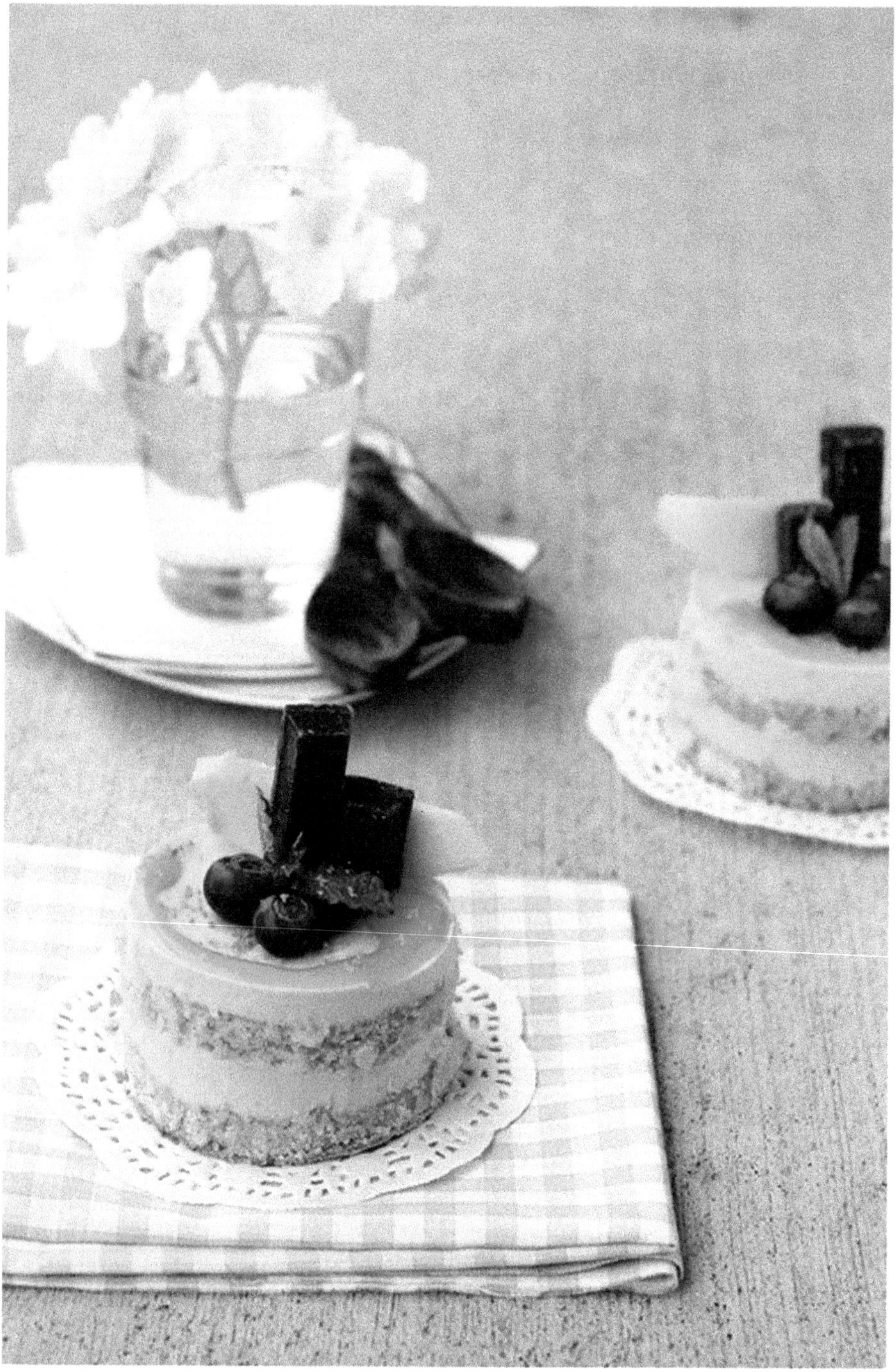

Lightning Source UK Ltd.
Milton Keynes UK
UKHW020705310521
384670UK00006B/72

9 781802 775020